EVERYTHING ABOUT ANTIPHOSPHOLIPID SYNDROME (APS)

A Complete Guide For Patients, Caregivers, And Healthcare Professionals - Causes, Symptoms, Diagnosis, Treatment, Coping Strategies, And More

DR. CADE JOSUE

Table of Contents

DISCLAIMER

The information provided in this book is for general informational purposes only. It is not intended as medical advice, diagnosis, or treatment.

The content of this book should not be considered a substitute for professional medical advice. Readers should consult with a qualified healthcare provider for diagnosis and treatment of any medical conditions they have.

While every effort has been made to ensure the accuracy and completeness of the information presented, the author makes no representations or warranties of any kind, express or implied, about the completeness, accuracy, reliability, suitability, or availability with respect to the information, contained in this book.

The author disclaims any responsibility for any loss or damage resulting from reliance on the information provided in this book. References to individuals, products, websites, organizations, or other names are for informational purposes only and do not imply endorsement.

By reading this book, readers acknowledge that they are responsible for their own health decisions and should seek appropriate medical advice when necessary.

ABOUT THIS BOOK

This book titled "Everything About Antiphospholipid Syndrome (APS)" provides comprehensive insights into numerous aspects of this intricate autoimmune disorder, making it an essential reference for medical practitioners, researchers, and patients. The initial segment establishes a strong groundwork by presenting an all-encompassing synopsis of APS, its historical milieu, and the progressive advancements in treatment and investigation. This establishes the foundation for an exhaustive examination of the syndrome's complexities.

An essential component addressed in this book is comprehension of the fundamental mechanisms and catalysts of APS, encompassing an exploration of the risk factors and causative elements that contribute to its onset.

This fundamental understanding is essential for the development of focused interventions and preventative measures. Subsequently, this book provides a comprehensive delineation of the varied symptoms and clinical presentations that are linked to APS, thereby enabling prompt identification and intervention.

A substantial segment of this book is devoted to the diagnostic process, providing clarification on the diverse tests and criteria that are employed to validate APS. This section is critical for improving the precision of diagnoses and guaranteeing suitable treatment.

Additionally, this book clarifies the various categories of antiphospholipid antibodies that are implicated in the development of APS, providing valuable perspectives on their clinical importance and ramifications for the treatment of patients.

This book further explores the interconnections between APS and various health conditions, including hematological disorders, skin disorders, neurological disorders, pregnancy, thrombosis, and stroke. Every chapter in this book offers a comprehensive comprehension of the intricate ways in which APS presents itself in various organ systems, thereby informing clinicians on how to customize patient care and maximize results.

Furthermore, the extensive scope of coverage includes emerging treatment modalities, immunomodulatory therapies, pharmacological interventions, and treatment options for APS. Furthermore, the publication underscores the significance of implementing lifestyle management techniques to alleviate complications associated with APS and enhance the overall well-being of individuals affected.

"Everything About Antiphospholipid Syndrome (APS)" serves as a seminal work in the medical literature, facilitating evidence-based practice, bridging knowledge gaps, and equipping individuals impacted by APS with resources and information to make well-informed decisions and adopt a holistic approach to management.

CHAPTER ONE

Antiphospholipid Syndrome (APS): An Overview

Antiphospholipid Syndrome (APS), alternatively referred to as Hughes Syndrome, is a blood-based autoimmune disorder distinguished by the presence of antiphospholipid antibodies (aPL).

Phospholipids, a class of fat molecules whose function is vital to blood coagulation, cell signaling, and other physiological processes, are inadvertently targeted by these antibodies.

Antibodies that target phospholipids may increase the likelihood of thrombosis, an anomalous formation of blood clots, in addition to causing complications that impact multiple organ systems.

Comprehension Of The Antiphospholipid Syndrome (APS)

Antiphospholipid syndrome (APS) is distinguished by the presence of three principal categories of antiphospholipid antibodies: anti-β2GPI, lupus anticoagulant (LA), and anticardiolipin antibodies (aCL). The antibodies in question interfere with the regular operation of phospholipids, resulting in an elevated propensity for the formation of blood clots. Furthermore, aPL has the potential to disrupt a multitude of cellular mechanisms, resulting in inflammation as well as harm to vital organs and blood vessels.

Categorization

A primary occurrence of APS or its co-occurrence with other autoimmune disorders, such as systemic lupus erythematosus (SLE), are both possible. When APS manifests alongside another autoimmune disorder, this co-occurrence is known as secondary APS. Primary APS denotes instances in which APS is the only autoimmune disorder that is present.

The Diagnosis Is As Follows:

A combination of laboratory testing and clinical evaluation is required to diagnose APS. The diagnosis is guided by criteria set forth by the International Society on Thrombosis and Haemostasis (ISTH), which stipulate the presence of a minimum of one clinical event (e.g., pregnancy complications or thrombosis) and two or more positive laboratory tests for aPL spaced at least 12 weeks apart.

Factors Contributing To And Posing A Risk For Antiphospholipid Syndrome

Autoimmune Processes:

Although the precise etiology of APS is unknown, it is hypothesized that environmental triggers and genetic predisposition are involved. It is hypothesized that immune system dysregulation is the cause of antiphospholipid antibody production, which subsequently results in the development of autoimmunity.

Contributing Genetic Factors:

There may be genetic predispositions that contribute to the development of APS. An illustration of this can be seen in the association of particular gene mutations with the immune system and blood clotting pathways with the onset of APS.

Environmental Stimuli:

Anxieties, hormonal fluctuations, medications, and specific aspects of lifestyle are examples of environmental factors that may exacerbate or initiate APS in susceptible individuals. It has been hypothesized that infections, specifically viral infections such as Epstein-Barr virus and cytomegalovirus, could potentially initiate APS.

Risk Elements:

The following factors increase the likelihood of developing APS:

• A familial predisposition to autoimmune disorders (APS)

• Female gender (APS is more prevalent among females)

• A prior diagnosis of additional autoimmune disorders, including systemic lupus erythematosus

Cessation Of Smoking

• Specific pharmaceuticals, including hormonal therapies and certain anti-epileptic drugs

Clinical Manifestations and Symptoms of Antiphospholipid Syndrome (APS)

Thrombosis Occurs When:

A high risk of thrombosis, which can develop in both veins and arteries across the body, is one of the defining characteristics of APS. Deep vein thrombosis (DVT) in the lower extremities, pulmonary embolism (PE), transient ischemic attacks (TIAs), myocardial infarctions (heart attacks), and strokes are all frequent sites of thrombosis. Life-threatening thrombotic events in APS necessitate immediate medical intervention.

Obstetric Complications:

There is an elevated likelihood that pregnant women who have APS will develop complications including preeclampsia, recurrent miscarriages, fetal growth restriction, and preterm birth. The compromised placental blood flow caused by thrombosis and inflammation gives rise to these complications.

Additional Clinical Presentations:

Beyond pregnancy complications and thrombosis, APS has the potential to induce an extensive array of additional clinical manifestations, which encompass:

• Neurological manifestations, including but not limited to migraines, seizures, cognitive decline, and motor dysfunction

• Dermatological presentations, including digital ischemia, livedo reticularis (lace-like dermatitis), and ulceration

Cardiovascular complications include cardiomyopathy and abnormalities of the heart valves.

• Renal complications, including glomerulonephritis and renal artery thrombosis

• Hematological irregularities, including hemolytic anemia and thrombocytopenia (low platelet count)

Clinical Presentation Variable:

Clinical manifestations of APS can differ significantly between those who are affected. Recurrent thrombotic events may manifest in some individuals as asymptomatic episodes, whereas in others, they may be accompanied by a multifaceted clinical course that encompasses various organ systems. Moreover, the intensity of symptoms may vary gradually, alternating between phases of improvement and worsening. In individuals with APS, early detection and appropriate management are crucial for enhancing prognoses and decreasing the likelihood of complications.

CHAPTER TWO

Diagnosis

Antiphospholipid Syndrome (APS) is a multifaceted autoimmune disorder distinguished by the existence of antiphospholipid antibodies (aPL), which induce thrombosis (i.e., blockages in the bloodstream) and potentially complicate pregnancy. To thoroughly examine the concepts you have presented:

1. Clinical Requirements:

• APS is typically diagnosed using a combination of clinical and laboratory criteria. Vascular thrombosis, including pulmonary embolism (PE) and deep vein thrombosis (DVT), as well as pregnancy complications such as recurrent miscarriages, stillbirths, or preterm births caused by severe preeclampsia or placental insufficiency, are clinical criteria.

• A variety of blood vessels, including veins, arteries, and minor vessels, are susceptible to thrombosis.

2. Laboratory Requirements:

Laboratory analysis entails the identification of antiphospholipid antibodies (aPL) in the specimen's blood. Examples of typical exams include:

The lupus anticoagulant (LA) assay quantifies the existence of LA, an assay product that paradoxically elevates the likelihood of thrombosis.

• Anti-cardiolipin antibodies (aCL): Phospholipids found in cell membranes that target cardiolipin.

Anti-beta2-glycoprotein I antibodies (anti-β2GPI) are a class of antibodies that target the plasma protein β2-glycoprotein I.

• At least 12 weeks should pass between aPL testing repetitions to confirm persistent positivity.

3. Further Considerations:

• False-positive results can be caused by infections and medications, among other conditions; therefore, a meticulous interpretation of clinical and laboratory findings is necessary for diagnosis.

A diagnosis of APS may give rise to substantial treatment and management considerations, such as the implementation of anticoagulation therapy to avert thrombosis and interventions to provide pregnancy support for those afflicted.

Varieties Of Antiphospholipid Syndrome

1. Anticoagulant For Lupus (LA):

• LA interferes with in vitro coagulation assays as a prothrombotic antibody and is not a true anticoagulant.

• It elevates the likelihood of developing pregnancy complications, including recurrent miscarriages, and arterial and venous thrombosis.

2. Acl: Anti-Cardiolipin Antibodies

• A phospholipid found in cell membranes, cardiolipin, is the target of these antibodies; they are linked to an increased risk of thrombosis and pregnancy complications.

• Antibodies against ACLs are categorized as IgG, IgM, or IgA, with IgG isotypes being frequently regarded as more clinically significant.

3. Antibodies Against Beta2-Glycoprotein I (anti-β2GPI):

• B2-glycoprotein I, a plasma protein that forms complexes with negatively charged phospholipids, is the target of anti-β2GPI antibodies.

• In APS, these antibodies are strongly associated with pregnancy complications and thrombosis.

The Association Between APS And Pregnancy

1. Obstetric Complications:

• Acquired thrombophilia associated with adverse pregnancy outcomes is most frequently caused by APS.

• Recurrent miscarriages, stillbirths, preterm births resulting from severe preeclampsia or placental insufficiency, and additional complications including fetal growth restriction are among the complications that women with APS are more susceptible to.

• During pregnancy, thrombosis can further confound prognoses for both the mother and the fetus.

2. Organizational Management:

• A multidisciplinary approach is required for the management of APS during pregnancy; obstetricians, hematologists, and rheumatologists are all involved.

• To prevent thrombosis and enhance pregnancy outcomes, anticoagulation therapy with low molecular weight heparin (LMWH) may be prescribed as part of the treatment plan.

• It is critical to maintain vigilant observation of the health of both the mother and the fetus during pregnancy, employing techniques like Doppler ultrasound to evaluate fetal development and placental blood flow.

3. Counseling Before Conception:

• Before becoming expectant, women with APS should receive preconception counseling to optimize their health.

Medication adjustments, such as the transition from warfarin to LMWH, may be required to mitigate potential dangers to the developing embryo.

APS And Thromboembolism

1. The Study Of Pathophysiology:

• Thrombosis associated with APS is caused by the interaction of antiphospholipid antibodies with diverse coagulation system components.

• The precise mechanisms through which aPL induces thrombosis remain incompletely elucidated; however, they probably encompass platelet activation, endothelial dysfunction, and disruption of coagulation pathways.

2. Clinical Indications:

• Thrombosis in APS can impact venous and arterial circulation, resulting in a variety of clinical manifestations including limb ischemia, deep vein thrombosis, stroke, and myocardial infarction.

• Recurrent thrombotic events that manifest at atypical sites can pose diagnostic difficulties.

3. Prevention And Treatment:

• The cornerstone of treatment for thrombotic events in APS is anticoagulation therapy.

• For secondary thromboprophylaxis, long-term anticoagulation with vitamin K antagonists (e.g., warfarin) or direct oral anticoagulants (DOACs) is typically advised.

• Acute situations, including thrombotic events that occur during pregnancy or catastrophic APS, may require the administration of high-dose anticoagulation.

In brief, APS is a complex condition distinguished by pregnancy complications and/or thrombosis that are facilitated by antiphospholipid antibodies. A combination of clinical criteria and laboratory testing is required for diagnosis, whereas a comprehensive, patient-specific approach is necessary for management. A comprehensive comprehension of APS and its multifaceted elements is imperative to maximize patient care and outcomes.

CHAPTER THREE

Antiphospholipid Syndrome And Stroke

Stroke represents a substantial manifestation of APS and ranks among the most prevalent causes of morbidity and mortality among those affected. Ischemic stroke is the most common consequence of thrombosis in the cerebral vasculature that is associated with APS.

Thrombotic events in APS may manifest in either the arterial or venous systems; however, stroke is more frequently correlated with arterial thrombosis. By promoting endothelial dysfunction, platelet activation, and coagulation cascade activation, the presence of aPL in APS raises the risk of thrombosis. Strokes associated with APS frequently impact young people and can transpire even in the absence of conventional risk factors for stroke.

APS And Cardiovascular Health

Antiphospholipid Syndrome (APS) presents considerable obstacles to cardiovascular well-being on account of its prothrombotic behavior. A variety of cardiovascular complications, such as myocardial infarction (heart attack), coronary artery disease, and valvular abnormalities, are more likely to develop in individuals with APS. Myocardial infarction can be caused by thrombosis in the coronary arteries; for myocardial ischemia, arterial and microvascular thrombosis may also play a role. Moreover, inflammation and endothelial dysfunction associated with APS can worsen the advancement of atherosclerosis, thereby augmenting the likelihood of cardiovascular incidents. Individuals with APS must have their conventional cardiovascular risk factors, including hypertension and hyperlipidemia, effectively managed to reduce the likelihood of developing cardiovascular complications.

The APS And Renal Health

Renal health can be impacted by APS via multiple mechanisms, such as thrombotic microangiopathy, thrombosis of the renal artery, and nephropathy which is concomitant with hypertension and chronic kidney disease. The development of microthrombi within the renal microvasculature is thrombotic microangiopathy, which has the potential to cause renal ischemia and organ impairment. Thrombus in the renal artery may cause acute kidney damage or infarction of the kidney affected. Furthermore, progressive renal injury may result from hypertension associated with APS, thereby exacerbating the risk of developing chronic kidney disease. In patients with APS, early detection and treatment of renal complications are critical for preventing renal failure and preserving kidney function.

Atopic Pneumonia And Skin Disorders

Antiphospholipid Syndrome (APS) is frequently accompanied by skin manifestations, which may take the form of livedo reticularis, cutaneous ulceration, or non-specific dermatitis, among others. A lace-like pattern of reddish-blue discoloration of the skin, known as Livedo reticularis, is among the most distinctive dermatological manifestations of APS.

Vasospasm or thrombosis of a small vessel causes a disruption in blood flow, which induces this condition. Ischemia and necrosis of the affected tissue may result in thrombotic events, which may give rise to corneal ulceration. Individuals with APS may also develop non-specific rashes, including purpuric or erythematous lesions, as a result of underlying vascular pathology. Dermatological manifestations in APS may serve as crucial clinical markers for disease monitoring and management, as they frequently correlate with disease activity.

To summarise, Antiphospholipid Syndrome (APS) is a multifaceted autoimmune condition that is notably correlated with substantial rates of illness and death. It is imperative to comprehend the diverse systemic manifestations of APS, encompassing its ramifications on cardiovascular health, cutaneous disorders, stroke, and renal function, to implement efficacious interventions and preempt complications in those afflicted. To provide comprehensive care for patients with APS, a multidisciplinary approach involving rheumatologists, hematologists, neurologists, cardiologists, nephrologists, and dermatologists is frequently required.

Neurological Disorders And APS

APS has the potential to impact the nervous system, resulting in a range of neurological symptoms. The spectrum of symptoms encompasses moderate conditions such as cognitive impairment and migraines, as well as severe ailments like stroke and seizures. The following are frequent neurological disorders linked to APS:

1. A prominent cause of stroke among adolescents is APS. A cerebral artery clogging may result in ischemic stroke, a condition characterized by nutrient and oxygen deprivation in a specific region of the brain.

2. Transient Ischemic Attack (TIA): Occurring in the context of APS, TIAs, which are frequently called "mini-strokes," are caused by a transient disruption in cerebral blood flow. These conditions present themselves in the form of temporary neurological symptoms, including lethargy or challenges with articulation.

3. Cognitive dysfunction can manifest in patients with APS, manifesting as challenges with memory, concentration, and various other cognitive functions. This can have a substantial effect on quality of life and daily life.

4. Seizures: Epileptic seizures may manifest in individuals with APS, potentially attributable to stroke or other autoimmune response-related mechanisms.

5. Chorea: A rare movement disorder, APS-associated chorea is distinguished by abrupt, involuntary movements. Typically, the face and extremities are affected.

6. Headaches: Frequent neurological manifestations of APS include headaches, which are frequently compared to tension-type headaches or migraines.

The diagnosis of neurological involvement in antiphospholipid syndrome (APS) necessitates the integration of several diagnostic components: laboratory tests that validate the existence of antiphospholipid antibodies, clinical assessment, and neuroimaging studies (e.g., MRI or CT scans).

CHAPTER FOUR

Hematological Disorders And APS

Hematological manifestations are prevalent in APS and predominantly comprise disruptions in the process of blood coagulation. In addition to causing recurrent miscarriages and other pregnancy-related complications, these may cause venous and arterial thrombosis. Prominent hematological disorders that are linked to APS comprise:

1. Deep vein thrombosis (DVT) and pulmonary embolism (PE), in which blood clots develop in the vessels of the lower extremities and subsequently migrate to the lungs, are complications that are further exacerbated by APS.

2. Arterial thrombosis can manifest in the arteries as well, giving rise to various medical complications including myocardial   infarction

(heart attack), peripheral arterial thrombosis, and stroke.

3. Thrombocytopenia: Low platelet counts, a pathological state experienced by certain patients with APS, are possible complications. This may also elevate the likelihood of developing bleeding complications alongside thrombosis.

4. A prominent etiology of recurrent miscarriages, specifically during the second and third trimesters, is APS. This is frequently the result of thrombotic events in the uterine blood vessels leading to placental insufficiency.

5. Hemolytic anemia is a rare complication of APS that results in the premature destruction of red blood cells, thereby inducing symptoms such as fatigue, weakness, and other indications of anemia.

Potential Therapies For APS

Preventing thrombotic events, managing associated symptoms, and minimizing pregnancy-related complications are the goals of APS management. Typical treatment strategies consist of:

1. Anticoagulation therapy is the fundamental approach to managing APS, which entails the administration of anticoagulant medications to inhibit the formation of blood clots. This may include direct oral anticoagulants (DOACs) or oral anticoagulants (warfarin) such as apixaban or rivaroxaban. As an initial treatment for acute thrombosis, heparin may be administered.

2. In addition to anticoagulants, antiplatelet agents such as aspirin may be prescribed to patients with APS who have experienced arterial thrombosis or who have substantial cardiovascular risk factors.

3. Immunosuppressive Therapy: To suppress the autoimmune response in patients with refractory APS or severe autoimmune manifestations, immunosuppressive medications such as rituximab, azathioprine, or corticosteroids may be considered.

4. Pregnant women diagnosed with APS necessitate specialized management to mitigate the risk of complications during pregnancy. This may entail the concurrent administration of low-dose aspirin and anticoagulant therapy (typically low molecular weight heparin), in addition to vigilant monitoring throughout the duration of pregnancy.

5. The management of cardiovascular risk factors in patients with APS requires lifestyle modifications including quitting smoking, engaging in regular physical activity, and maintaining a healthy weight. Patients should also maintain adequate hydration and avoid prolonged

immobility, particularly during lengthy flights or periods of inactivity.

6. Consistent Monitoring: Anticoagulation levels must be routinely monitored in patients with APS, in addition to conducting screenings for cardiovascular risk factors and complications including hypertension, diabetes, and hyperlipidemia.

7. Patient education concerning the characteristics of APS, the significance of adhering to prescribed medications, and the ability to identify symptoms indicative of thrombosis or pregnancy complications is critical. Additionally, counseling and support groups can be beneficial resources for patients coping with the difficulties of having APS.

To summarise, the treatment of APS necessitates a comprehensive multidisciplinary strategy that includes the administration of anticoagulant therapy, immunosuppression, adjustments to one's lifestyle, and specialized pregnancy management care. While minimizing the risk of complications, many patients with APS can lead fulfilling lives with the assistance of appropriate treatment and monitoring.

Summary

In summary, Antiphospholipid Syndrome (APS) poses an intricate and diverse obstacle within the domain of autoimmune disorders. Antiphospholipid antibodies are the defining characteristic of this condition, which is accompanied by an extensive spectrum of symptoms including thrombosis, complications during pregnancy, neurological impairments, and dermatological problems. Notwithstanding substantial advancements in comprehending the pathophysiology and clinical management of APS, it continues to be a diagnosis laden with uncertainties and ever-changing nuances.

A multidisciplinary approach is required for the effective management of APS, which includes the collaboration of obstetricians, hematologists, rheumatologists, and other specialists. Anticoagulation therapy is the fundamental approach to preventing thrombotic events, whereas targeted interventions target particular manifestations, such as complications related to the nervous system or abortion. Furthermore, current research initiatives aim to elucidate the complex mechanisms that underlie APS to develop innovative therapeutic approaches and individualized treatment plans.

In addition to medical interventions, patient education, and support are crucial components in enabling individuals with APS to effectively manage its intricacies and achieve personal satisfaction. Additional measures such as awareness campaigns and advocacy endeavors serve to augment public comprehension and cultivate a nurturing atmosphere for individuals impacted by this particular condition.

Fundamentally, although APS presents considerable obstacles, continuous progress in research and clinical application provides optimism regarding enhanced results and quality of life for those contending with this enigmatic syndrome.

THE END